MIDWIFE
and Other Poems on Caring

by
Marilyn Krysl

with preface and introduction by
Jean Watson, PhD, RN, FAAN
Dean and Professor of Nursing
Associate Director, Department of Nursing
Director of the Center for Human Caring
University of Colorado Health Sciences Center
School of Nursing
Denver, Colorado

Pub. No. 21-2286

National League for Nursing • New York

Second Printing

The views expressed in this book reflect those of the authors and do not necessarily reflect the official views of the National League for Nursing.

ISBN 0-88737-448-4

Manufactured in the United States of America

CONTENTS

Preface and Introduction—Jean Watson

Celebration of the Body 1
The Womb is the Body's Most Powerful Muscle 3
Feet 4
Skin 6

Food as Power/Power as Food 9
Home Call: Mother and Child 11
Mother with Newborn, Commerce City, Colorado 13
Connie: The Greenhouses 15

Violence and Dignity 17
Quadriplegic: The Bath 19
Thread 21
Burn Patient 23

Moral Baptism 25
Neonatal ICU: Mother and Child 27
Burn Unit: Baptist 29
The Other 31

Metaphysics 33
Sunshine Acres Living Center 35
There Is No Such Thing As The Moment Of Death 37
The Birthing Room 38
Midwife 40

PREFACE

Center For Human Caring

The Center for Human Caring was established in 1986 by the University of Colorado School of Nursing. It's overall mission is to explore new ways of advancing the art and science of human caring knowledge, ethics, and clinical practice in the fields of nursing and health sciences. Specifically, the center is designed to foster the study, teaching, and practice of human caring by drawing upon the underdeveloped connections between nursing science caring theory and knowledge from the humanities, and applying the rapidly growing scientific knowledge base which expands the relationship between human caring, health, and healing outcomes. Center efforts range from specific curricular activities in nursing and health sciences to piloting and researching new educational practice models of excellence in human caring and healing. The center offers public and professional forums and institutes, hosts resident scholars from diverse backgrounds, sponsors interdisciplinary programs and projects, and disseminates information through formal and informal educational programs and official publications.

Marilyn Krysl is a prize-winning poet and author who was artist in residence in the Center for Human Caring during the 1987–1988 academic year. During her residency, she was commissioned to engage in the many activities and lived experiences of the world of faculty, students, patients, and families. The experiences took place in settings that ranged from specific institutional clinical settings—such as the burn unit, neonatal intensive care, cardiac unit, home and community visits, senior citizen units—to nighttime birthing experiences with nurse midwives.

INTRODUCTION TO *MIDWIFE AND OTHER POEMS ON CARING*

The profession of nursing is in major transition, struggling to define and redefine itself in the midst of quantum changes in science, society, and the health care (medical-cure) system. As nursing emerges as a health discipline in its own right, it needs to find its own language, its own voice. Only then will nursing come of age as the health and human caring profession it is destined to become. As it does so, it will have the confidence of its own voice, and stand on its own philosophy, theories, ethics and human science dimensions that integrate all ways of knowing—from the empirical to the metaphysical. Its human caring practices and methods of discovery can then be confidently grounded in ancient and timeless traditions, as well as the latest advanced artistic and scientific human caring-healing modalities. In order to get there, we have to see anew the art and science of human caring in nursing, to shed light where there has been institutional and scientific darkness.

Maxine Greene points out in her recent work (1988) that what society perhaps needs at this point in history is to break from our mere routine, the "cotton wool" of habit, to seek alternative ways of being (as well as knowing and doing), to find new ways of achieving freedom. Such a challenge is particularly poignant for the contemporary world of medicine and nursing, which is often swallowed in an absence of care, in the midst of economic priorities, overwhelming shortages of professional nurses, and a surging hospital industry and techno-cure preoccupation. Quoting Foucault, Greene (1988) points out there is little evidence of a desire to think about what we are doing—little evidence of thought about the consequences for the human mind and spirit. As Foucault stated..."thought is freedom in relation to what one does, the motion by which one detaches oneself from it, establishes it as an object, and reflects upon it as a problem" (Foucault in Greene, 1988, p.2). In addition Greene emphasizes the concept of human consciousness, a moment of being, that calls upon language in order to speak in one's own voice...to overcome, to find and experience freedom, along with a new consciousness in relation to what one does.

Marilyn Krysl's poetry provides a new language and a new voice for nursing's quest to seek alternative ways of being in relation to human caring and healing in the midst of a world emphasizing body physical fixes, techno-cure, and costs at the expense of the changing human consciousness. Her work is a voice by which we can capture caring moments of being; sing a hymn of meditation in a language which allows us to detach ourselves from the harsh world of institutions and establish the human caring occasion as a transcendent way of being; an opportunity to reflect upon the integration of mind-body-spirit; of the full engagement of the human self and human spirit in caring and healing. This collection of her works helps us to see anew the full knowing which comprises nursing science, practice, and education. The poetry helps us to experience the empirical, aesthetic, personal, intuitive, ethical, and metaphysical. All of these dimensions are captured within a new consciousness of moral as well as political choices and consequences for nursing and society.

In summary, Marilyn Krysl helps us to push away the rock of apathy, of disinterest, of lassitude, and experience and feel the warm rays of light and energy that shine forth from the human spirit of caring embedded in nursing's most seemingly mundane acts. This work helps nursing to turn toward some new possibilities to find another language that provides it with its own voice. Therefore we are able to see new ways of being in the world of clinical care; to reach beyond, toward what is not yet in our awakened consciousness, but perhaps ought to be, must be, if nursing is to awaken to its own spirit and come alive for a new order.

REFERENCE

Greene, M. (1988). *The dialectic of freedom.* New York: Teachers College Press.

MIDWIFE
and Other Poems on Caring

CELEBRATION OF THE BODY

Our bodies are our world. They are both end and means for us. In the body we live and move and have our being. In the body we have our comedy and our tragedy, our joys and sorrows. We recognize the body as our instrument, the instrument through which we live out our existence. In caring for others and in accepting care from others we experience the spiritual community which can only take place in this world, in the flesh.

"The Womb Is the Body's Most Powerful Muscle" celebrates the intensity of a mother's body knowledge at the moment just before birth. "Feet" presents a comic view of ourselves and our physical being. "Skin" rejects the Puritan ethic of denying, subduing, and suppressing the body, and treats the skin, that medium through which we carry on human communication with each other, as imminently worthy of praise. The poem ventures even further afield, arguing that touch is not only essential to our physical well being, but that this tactile form of communication, or lack of it, has important psychological and social effects and profound political consequences as well.

The Womb is the Body's Most Powerful Muscle

The woman has become a red

intensity. She has brought all that is necessary
down the passageway as far as the central
hall, and now see how she

listens. She stands at the
threshold, listening around the oval
opening, pressed out just so far by the new being's
crown. As a lifter of weights
listens for the collection of her
forces, this woman listens
around a dome of bone
for the sound of a drop of water on the stone

threshold. Do not
disturb her. Any
moment now,
that drop of water

will fall.

Feet

They are the last to leave
the womb. The woman feels two little fins
fluttering, this is the last time

you fly. Now they're
weights, they keep you
down to earth. Flat as the land
you stand on, they go *flop, flop,* a pair of
turbot, each in its separate tureen,
and instead of a pair some of us have two lefts
and we put them in our mouths, and they're not

pretty. You never saw your father
without socks. Now when your lover undresses
the foot is the one appendage you don't want to look at,
to touch. Feet are

indecent, certainly unfit for
jewelry, and not exotic—just
odd. Likely candidates for dropped
tins of tomatoes, something to step on while
dancing. Even the Chinese failed to find
any grace in them, wrapped them in bandages
and tried to kill them. And the prima ballerina
tucks one under her wing like a flamingo
and tries to sublimate the other into her leg
and if she's good we believe for split seconds at a time

that they don't exist at all. All around the world
women stand at their mirrors, sighing, "If only
we could end at the ankles." They get

cold, they lack any interesting
orifices, all you can do is make clumsy
passes under the table
and like two great brooches grandmother gave you
you can't give them away. White elephants,
they belong in a museum,
keep them in a glass coffin
and charge admission. When you walk
slap, slap, they remind you you're not going
anywhere. And when you feel shame and look down
they seem to confirm it. *It's a miracle,* they say,
that once or twice you managed to dance, and they

smell. And when you finally lie down alone the last time
there they are at the bottom of the bed,
the only thing left upright. Tombstones.
Feet are the last thing you see

before your eyes close.

Skin

Because skin is the first organ
    to form in the womb, and first things
    are of first importance.

Because skin is the largest
    organ—an adult's skin
    weighs six pounds
    and stretched out
    covers eighteen square feet

Because there is more of it to attend to
    than anything else

Because the skin's resilience
    can only be experienced

Because it feels superior by far
    to silk or challis

    and in addition is lovely
    to look at, nothing by Cardin
    comes close to it

Because it's the organ with which we experience wind,
    which most loves water,

Because it's the organ through which we begin
    to discover each other,

because, because, because, because,
    and for all these good reasons

hurry out and touch someone now!

Delay in this matter
is not
a good idea,
you have delayed too long
already, your suffering brothers and sisters
are waiting, you can hardly expect them to wait
much longer, and remember
when you touch another
person,

the skin
gives off a chemical
which makes them
and you
feel better
more alert
more cheerful
more willing to take chances
more open to new experience
more generally obstreperously intent on securing
the greatest good for everybody
and more likely to say NO to the MX
and YES to the levy for the public schools

After all, it's
the organ

through which we take in
the light we give out

FOOD AS POWER/POWER AS FOOD

Power as we know it, in relations between people, is as basic as food. It is like food in its effect on us. Using our power to give to another person is like feeding that person. Taking what someone else offers is like eating. Many are the ways in which we can feed each other, and all of us flourish and are at our best when we manage not to share power but to share in it. When we feed and are fed by each other, power becomes the fluid essence of the universe, that which is in us all and which belongs to no one.

But food and "feeding" are sometimes used as tools of aggression in power relationships. On a global scale rich nations (we call them "world powers") are in a position to give or refuse food and other kinds of care to poor nations. National governments take a similar position in regard to their constituents. And on an individual level a parent has the power to give or refuse food and care to a child.

Caregivers, however, understand their relationships with patients are reciprocal. No one is human alone. A patient wanting to die may be kept alive by means of technology, "maintained" in a physical state technically referred to as "alive." But this person does not "live." The will to live, the choice to live, is a personal one.The patient and no one else possesses this will, this choice. Thus a caregiver is continuously assessing the patient's perception of his or her own will. The caregiver has to feel, to intuit the patient's attitude toward self, toward the caregiver, and toward the relationship between the two of them. What the caregiver must do then is somehow to remind the patient of that will, call up the desire to be, to heal, to recover, to begin to live, to thrive. The caregiver must, in a sense, remind the patient of his or her own dignity. When the patient once again assumes this dignity, the caregiver must recognize it and allow it.

The caregiver's "power" then is the power to bring forth what the patient already possesses: free choice and personal desire.

In this situation power is not an exclusive possession of one at the expense of another but is instead an atmosphere in which two become a community, become "one." "Home Call: Mother and Child" attempts to articulate how deeply ingrained in us is the habit of perceiving each other in terms of power potential. In this poem I was interested in articulating three situations: first, how the patient may perceive the caregiver in an oversimplified, stereotyped way as one in a position to dispense services, as a person with power over the patient; second, how the patient may perceive herself as weak, dependent on the caregiver; and third, how the caregiver is aware that this is the patient's perception, and how she must include this knowledge in her imminent decisions. "Mother with Newborn, Commerce City, Colorado" delineates the complex, imaginative, and compassionate perceptions of a caregiver faced with a difficult, perhaps "impossible" task. And "Connie: The Greenhouses" makes clear that the caregiver is not simply a professional but is also a human being, a part of the human equation. She too is a person multiple and varied, complicated and needy. In this poem the caregiver who "feeds" others is also "fed" by them, and she knows, understands and welcomes this, and recognizes this exchange is an essential fact of the process of caring. This poem attempts to clearly lay out the ways in which the relationship between the caregiver, Connie, and her patient, Castenga, is a mutual one, how their giving and receiving extends beyond the two of them out into the community, and how truly satisfying to the caregiver is this multiplied mutuality.

Home Call: Mother and Child

There's so little here: one table,
not laden, one blind
shut. One bulb
hung straight down. One woman,

not well (that look
of someone who won't talk
because they've been beaten
so the bruises don't show), and one

boy, dancing over, no
diaper, eager for the coin
of candy you lay in his
hand. He leans into your

yellow dress, reaching up,
a tendril attaching, lifting
out of the dark, unfurling
his last leaf. She watches him

watch you,
                    you with a house
she imagines half glass, where light
pours in, and everything
is already paid for: your

dress, the shine of health you wear
as though you own it, the look
of wealth, and (this too is
visible) the knowhow

to make the right phone calls,
calls to those, who, when you call,
will do what you say, pay
what you tell them, when

and to whom. You, she imagines,
who have at least two
of everything, you lift her son
to your yellow breast, that

well lighted place, where the air's
clean, and you don't
hate yourself, waiting in line
to pay for a sack of potatoes

you can't afford. She watches him
cling to you, she waits to see
what you will do: you who
have things, you who can

do things, you who can do
what you choose to, you
who can do something for them,
if you choose to, a little something

or nothing.

Mother with Newborn, Commerce City, Colorado

Crib in the corner: each cry
juts up,
                    lightning
across the nerves. You

stand and stare out, a woman
so thin you seem
just more of the dimness

in this room five hundred feet
from the highway, where a Diesel
reams the air, going aggressively

west, away from here.
                              In Renoir's painting
Maternity, the mother looks like the wife
of a burgher, buxom, filling with pleasure
as the baby sucks, indolent
and fat, a cherub

feeding on the Infinite. The two
seemed one complete figure, so
full this babe and breast
the whole just might
burst. The first time
I saw this painting, I just stood there
and stared, peering in at that
shrine, that psalm of milk, that worship
of food.

                    Somewhere there's art
and its history. Here in Commerce City
what there is is obscurity. Little
is the light you see by, what little money
there is goes for coffee,

and how *can* you feed a baby
when you're hungry, especially when you've
always been hungry, as far back as you can
remember, lying in the crib, nothing
inside you but your own
insides,
so that you swaddled yourself
in your own screaming, that sound
like cloth being ripped again
and again,
that tearing
scaring you so you cried
harder, trying to comfort yourself
with the thing that consumed you

and no one came. How can I presume to tell you

you should feed your baby. You of little
flesh, afraid this flowery creature
will eat

what's left of you. You
who aren't sure you can manage
the eyes
too new to focus, the tiny hands
like sepals, and the
asking, the aching, the empty

mouth—more
weight

added to the uncertainty
of your own body. You
who were not fed

and now cannot believe.

Connie: The Greenhouses

Commerce City, grit
thickening the air, and you can't
get a job here, not

much of one, and if you do it'll eventually
kill you. I'm hungry. Here
you forget to eat, or you don't

want to, the beauty
of an apple or good bread seems not to
fit here, and you fall

into hypnosis: the drone of the
Interstate is the sound of
monotony. Notice how the word sounds like

poverty, and is. The rooves of the greenhouses
glitter like rhinestones, and beyond, the tinny lids
of shacks, where, in the dimness,

new babies
are sprouting. I know where to go. The dogs
know me now. Little boys

take my hands, their chatter
the sound color would make
if it spoke. In their mouths my name

is a green blurr,
a whirr in blue air, as though I too
have come far, leaving behind

an equator, bringing what I could
carry. Here at the door
those good smells: Castenga

will feed me—posole,
fahitas, frijoles—braid
straight down her spine, and the radio

on. Castenga's orange skirt is the light
        we see by, babies a covey of quail
                at her feet. Now she holds out

the new one, talking bright talk
        to this boy, the bulb
                of a lily, fat with its

juices. She is proud of this
        fifth one, though her veins ache, and her
                feet hurt, and there's not enough sleep

to go around. How he
        glistens, this new one, oiled
                and round as an olive, and already,

pinned to his nightshirt, a silver
        medal
                against evil. For there are evil

spirits, I too believe this, I have
        seen them strike the living down
                again and again, and before their

prime. You do what you can
        against evil, you feed those who
                fight it, you give them a bed and your

blankets, what talismans against it
        you have. Now I take this new boy
                against me. This is how it always

is here: someone offering me
        something good
                to eat or to hold.

VIOLENCE AND DIGNITY

Just as food is basic to power, so is human dignity. It is at once both as present as a steel girder and vulnerable as a butterfly's wing. It can be a powerful personal tool and it can be destroyed by a casual remark. It can be snuffed out by physical violence and by both overt and subtle, insinuating forms of psychological violence. We can recognize and affirm dignity in ourselves, and deny or affirm it in others. This power to deny or affirm is not necessarily limited by class, race, or economic status. Any individual can acknowledge and respect or ignore and deny the dignity of another.

Dignity is essential to health. Without it we do not flourish. Without respect for and attention to it, an injured person may not heal. In "Quadriplegic: The Bath" I have tried to show not just the absence of violence but the active affirmation of another's human being. In the poem the caregiver openly and directly concedes power to the quadriplegic, confirming his dignity, saluting the virility he still possesses. In "Thread" the caregiver acknowledges Wiona's importance by honoring her last request and recognizing Wiona's final gesture as ritual. Wiona, who is dying, threads the needle, honors the life cycle. Honoring this moment, the caregiver affirms Wiona's dignity. "Burn Patient" attempts to imagine how devastating the loss of dignity as a result of psychological violence can be.

Quadriplegic: The Bath

"You'll feel like
new," I said, keeping things
breezy, as though we all know
how getting clean feels
good, no one in their
right mind
would refuse it, because he looked
like he just might file
a dissenting opinion. Which he could

do. Though he couldn't
get up and go—*bye, sugar buns,*
I'm walkin' out on you—which is
what he'd have

liked to do. He leaned
back then, the old stinker, like Caesar
in his chariot, and let me see his
penis, that loose fold
of flag that would not
fly again,
and said, "M'am, you seem to have
the wrong man. I don't require either your services
or your opinions." I could see

how indeed
neither service nor opinion
would be of the slightest
use to him. "O.K., all
right," I said, hand across
forehead, in mock
shock, letting him know the sharpness of the male
was in him still. "O.K.," I said, "I get
the picture." And I turned and was
going, leaving him the privacy
he had once, like a general,

commanded. "Aw
shit," he said, and with a wide sweep
drew me in. "You'll catch hell
if you don't do me. Anyway,
I stink. Come on with your
scrub brush."

So I knelt beside the water
the orderlies had set him in
and began to bathe him.

Thread

1.

The anesthesia wears off
and I watch her feel along the edges of light
for an opening. She

sees. She remembers
who she is—Wiona,
a woman who likes to be
up and about! She sits up quick,

then lies back
down: sits up again, slowly this time,

and only part way.

2.

She dreams the tree outside her kitchen, hung
with starlings. Fat,
like speckled fruits they weigh the limbs,

dark plums.

3.

She
loops thread
under and up, over and along
a hem. Each stitch is a

snake, its tail
in the mouth of the
next one. That stitch
that goes on

and on. But she's
out of thread. I say I'll
get some, at the Seven
Eleven. I move through the halls, the

wheelchairs, out past
pedestrians, traffic, the everlasting
repetitions. Those birds won't
fly, I think, until I

get back. And they
don't. She opens
the spool, unwinds a length, and I think

how we're always
beginning again
and again, as Wiona, dying,

insists on
filling a needle
with new thread.

Burn Patient

I did it
myself. That

I remember. Buying
gasoline in a
can, getting ready
in my room—I knew that dress
my father liked

still fit. I could hear his voice,
rising out of the past. "It's got to be
done," he'd said. "It's the only thing
to do." I took

a long drink
of water. Light
lay in a bar across
the floor, sacred cloth, laid out
before me. I put on the

dress then. That
I remember. And I remember
pouring the gas
on my belly

and crying. It seemed
sad, the water
so sweet, that striking a match
was the only thing

to do. But that didn't
stop me. *It's got to be done,* that's
what I remember. What I can't

remember now
is why.

MORAL BAPTISM

Medical ethics are in flux. Technology now makes it possible to keep people alive in circumstances which were previously extremely unlikely. At the same time, by extending life, technology also increases the possible and probable duration of pain. This situation, brought about by technological advance, raises ethical issues. Does a fetus have rights? What rights do prospective parents have? Should individuals be allowed to choose to die? Should caregivers assist them in this process? Is an injured person competent to make life and death decisions? Is it the obligation of caregivers to treat patients and to preserve life even against patients' wishes?

These questions deeply disturb us. They affect us all, and they have an especially profound effect on both caregivers and patients. I have not tried to answer these questions, but I have tried to probe divergent points of view on some of these issues. The poems in this section do not by any means exhaust possible points of view. Such a survey would itself constitute a book. Rather these poems isolate and articulate only a few of the more obvious attitudes toward ethical issues. "Neonatal ICU: Mother and Child" articulates one new mother's reaction to her baby's situation at one moment in time. "Burn Unit: Baptist" presents one person's reaction to extreme pain. And "The Other" attempts to clarify the complicated and emotionally difficult matter of psychological separation between caregivers and those who receive care.

Neonatal ICU: Mother and Child

Now I see I made it
for them. This creaturous
thing, thighs—if you can

call that a thigh—the size
of my thumb. Head turned
to one side, strapped
down. Tubes

in the openings. Tape
over the place of the penis,
tape with a slit in it

where the mouth should be. And all around,

machinery. I've made
a thing for them, not good,
a dangle of a thing
not good for it, or me. But

useful. See how it keeps the machines
going. See how the needles
record, how the tubes
thrust in and don't

stop. Though now it lies
still, a pincer
might pick it up by a

corner, flip it
over, drop it under
that light. Day

or night, you never know
which, or when, someone in a
white coat

comes with tools you don't
recognize, and then
examine! examine!

this cut off
bit of me,
that might, if I'd been smart,
have been a boy.

If I'd been
alone
I'd have held it
to make it feel good

while it was dying. Then
I'd have gone to the
woods—if there
were woods—

and there
I'd have put it
back in the earth
it came from. Instead

I've made them a live thing
they can use
and use. I can tell you

what hell is: the thrum
and whine
of a machine

that doesn't break down.

Burn Unit: Baptist

These women say
it's pain I feel, but it's

the fire. How complete
it is, like the way they
describe God, when you're a
kid: *He is always*

with you. I am
everywhere
open
to His probing

fingers. It's never about to begin,
and it's never over. It's
now, and He never
sleeps, and you can't

walk away. Everything
stops, except
the fire: it's fire
that's everlasting. These women

keep me breathing, they
feed me through a tube, they
feed me and feed me and think they're doing

good—I see, through the blur
heat makes of the air
their conviction that theirs
is an act of

compassion. They think
they love me. What they
don't understand

is that feeding the fire
keeps it going. Once
you're burning

it goes on and on
until someone who can

puts the fire out.

The Other

When I watched them clip away the bandages
and unwrap the burned man, I envied them,
as he must have, their motion, bending
and snipping, turning and rehooking a tube

as they talked to him. Though he could not speak
and did not move, except when they moved
a part of him, one lifting a leg while another
clipped away gauze, there was a moment's

pause when his right hand opened, palm up,
quivering, he raised his right hand, as though
reaching for something just out of reach.
Now she'll take it in hers, I thought, the one

beside him, because she'd laid
her scissors aside. I watched her
stand and watch his hand fall back.
Though they spoke kindly, they were cheerfully

matter of fact, as though unpacking
supplies, as though soon he would rise, leave them
to the rest of the inventory. Oh they are wise,
I thought, these women, to wash him, to wrap him

but not to become too attached to him,
the other. For he will indeed leave them,
just as they imagine. He will leave them
alone, a changed man, one way or another.

METAPHYSICS

Caring for others takes place, so to speak, in the metaphysical realm. We cannot "see" this realm, but we experience it. Over and over I watched the caregiver and the person accepting care as they came to constitute one wholeness. When two of us enter into each other this way, willingly and receptively, transformation takes place. The gestalt of our separate beings loosens and vibrates. The material of our being and becoming begins to flow. We experience ourselves and each other as elemental substance. We experience the living field of our interconnectedness. And we are filled with energy, a living material, palpable, substantial. This energy is nearly visible in the air around us. It is as though we give off light.

These moments of transcendence are fascinating. They occurred again and again, each time flowering forth, a moment of intense energy, of very material presence. I felt I was witnessing the invisible made substance. I was witnessing the spirit made flesh. The poems which follow try to articulate this transforming experience.

In "Sunshine Acres Living Center" two people enter each other's life histories and phenomenal fields. Doing so, they are transformed. No longer are they separate dancers: instead they have become a couple, one energy. They become fuller, richer, more substantial persons together in that moment. In "There Is No Such Thing As The Moment Of Death" a similar transformation takes place. The caregiver attending the dying man "hears" his death as the sound of her own blood. His death and her continuing are one process. In "The Birthing Room" I hoped to describe the atmosphere—charged, intense, and ecstatic—generated by the advent of birth, and to convey the spiritually transforming moment of one of life's most common and yet most amazing occasions. Finally, "Midwife" suggests the vast resources, the complexity, the intelligence, and power of the caregiver at work in the metaphysical realm.

Sunshine Acres Living Center

The first thing you see up ahead is Mr.
Polanski, wedged in the
arched doorway, like he means absolutely
to stay there, he who shouldn't
be here in the first place, put in here
by mistake, courtesy of that grandson
who thinks himself a hotshot, and too busy
raking in the dough to find time for an old
man. If Polanski had anyplace
to go, he'd be out
instantly, if he had any

money. Which he doesn't, but he does have
a sharp eye, and intends to stay in that
doorway, not missing
a thing, and waiting
for trouble. Which of course
will come. And could be
you—you're handy, you look
likely, you have

the authority. And
you're new here, another young
whippersnapper, doesn't know
ass from elbow, but has been given
the keys. Well he's

ready, Polanski. *Mr. Polanski, good
morning*—you say it in Polish,
which you learned a little of
when you were little, and your grandmother
taught you a little song about lambs, frisking
in a pen, and you danced a silly little dance
with your grandmother, while the two of you
sang. So you sing it

for him, here in the dim, institutional
light of the hallway, light which even you
find insupportable, because even those who just
work here, and can leave when their
shift ends, deserve light to
see by, and because it reminds you
of the light in the hallway
outside the room
where, when your grandmother
died, you were three thousand miles

away. So that you're singing the little song
and remembering the silly little dance
to console yourself, and to pay your grandmother
tribute, and to try to charm Polanski,

which you do: you sing, and Mr. Polanski,
he who had set himself against the doorjamb
to resist you, he who had made of himself
a fist, Mr. Polanski,
                    contentious, often
                    combative and always
                    and finally
                    inconsolable

hears that you know
the song. And he steps out
from the battlement
of the doorway, and begins to
shuffle

and sing along.

There Is No Such Thing
As The Moment Of Death

I work nights, and he was awake.
When he saw me, he said, "I'm not going to
make it." Well when they say that
they know. People can tell. You don't

argue with an expert. I wet the cloth
and bathed his face, but it didn't do him
good. So I took his hands in my two
and we held on. No one

was alone in that motion. The way water
is a part of itself, we were the going
until his hands went slack in mine.
Still I held on, some final acknowledgment

beginning its climb out of the body,
his skin resilient still, that shine
across a taut thing—then I saw it sag
and go flat. His body had a clearness

about it then, the clean weightlessness
of a crucible completely empty,
in which you hear the air ticking
against the glaze. Then I heard another

sound, like when you're a kid, holding
a shell to your ear, hearing
the ocean. I held on, and then I understood:
it was the sound of my own blood.

The Birthing Room

It's like stepping into a slow

elevator. You feel the pressure beginning to climb,
lifting the scale, the scissors, the basins, the clamps,
the light, the air and the white mound
of the mother, that muscle pulsing at the center

of the room. You have come into a room
that is rising, and you are round and lifting
off the round earth, flying a little, as you were
meant to, hovering over this sphere—labor—

You seem one with the nurse measuring the opening,
with the mother's sister whispering in her ear,
with the midwife waiting, calm in her blue gown—
and as you rise in the air with these women

the mother bears down. She bears down and the room
rises—oh but she feels she's about to fly off—
as though these three laid their hands on her flesh,
this clay—and said *ascend*. Now they kneel, they stand,

they lean over the mother, they lift their arms
like wings, they say soon. *Soon*
they croon, turning, looping over and around
the mother, and as they gather, as they turn

and wind and attend, as they bend to her
they touch her hand, her thigh, her hair,
talking to her the way you talk to a woman
in a room that is rising into the air.

Rising now like the sweep of an updraft,
rising now like the shouts of a crowd,
inevitable as bread in which the yeast
is good. The midwife says *I can see the crown*

and together now they lift the last distance,
and the room rises the last distance,
the midwife says *now, here, bear down*

and the mother cries out a great cry
and rises up amazed, like a flag suddenly unfurled,
rises, and pushes the child
                                        down,

down and out
into the world.

Midwife

Though I seem to wait
	I'm moving at the speed of light

Though I seem to stand by
	I'm running easily over the windswept grasslands
	to where the river divides the plains from the mountains

Though I seem to stand by
	I'm gathering the sweet and the bitter herbs
	in shade and in sunlight
	I'm digging out the bones of the lost animals
	embedded in the lakes of tar

Though I seem idle
	I'm releasing the father's fear into the wind,
	watching the wind disperse it

Though I seem idle
	I'm sending the mother the energy of the waves of the deep
	and of the shallow waters

Though I seem idle
	I'm traveling by night and by day, over earth and over sea
	to meet the new being

When I time the contractions
	I'm counting the sheeves of grain gathered in the mother's
	harvest

When I measure the opening
	I'm calculating the number of followers in the mother's
	fields

And when I touch the father's shoulder
	I'm singing the many names of the ancestors who overcame
	fear

When I seem to pause
I send light to the father, to the mother, to the older sister

When I seem to pause
I send light to those who will wash and wrap the new being

When I listen to the heartbeat of the new being coming
I hear the thud of the rapids upriver

When I listen to the heartbeat of the mother
I hear the tumbling of water down a great falls

When I lean forward, hands cupped for the head
I'm dividing the wind in the four directions

When I lean forward, hands cupped for the head
I'm gathering together the rain and the desert heat

And when at last I hold the head in my hands
I've hoisted the sun to the pinnacle of the heavens

When I hold the new being in my hands
I've brought the mother, father and child to the center of the eleven sacred circles

And when I lay the new being on the mother's breast
I'm sending the flocks of goats out to graze on the hillsides and in the valleys
I'm setting the fish loose at the headwaters of the rivers
I'm letting the birds go upward and out into the great migrations

When I clamp the cord in two places
I'm saying the child's two names,
one from the mother, one from the father

When I give the father the tool to cut the cord
I'm binding three people together
until the death of the last of the three

When I take the print of the new being's foot
I'm writing in the ancient alphabet the word just uttered

When I wait for the placenta
I'm spreading bleached linen on all the mattresses of darkness

And when it comes, when I examine the placenta
I'm sorting the particles and waves in the spectrum of light

And when my work is finished and I go from the place of birth
I walk out across the fields of the planets
into the spaces between the furthest stars

Marilyn Krysl is the author of five books of poetry (*Saying Things*, Abattoir Editions, University of Nebraska Press, 1978; *More Palomino, Please, More Fuchsia*, Cleveland State Poetry Center, 1980; *Diana Lucifera*, Shameless Hussy Press, 1983; *What We Have To Live With*, Teal Press, 1989; and *Midwife and Other Poems on Caring*, National League for Nursing, 1989) and two books of short stories (*Honey, You've Been Dealt A Winning Hand*, Capra Press, 1980; *Mozart, Westmoreland and Me*, Thunder's Mouth Press, 1985), as well as numerous essays, articles, and reviews. Her work has appeared in *The Atlantic*, *The Nation*, *The New Republic*, and many other journals, as well as in *O. Henry Prize Stories* and the *Pushcart Prize Anthology*. She has been the recipient of a grant from the National Endowment for the Arts, and in 1986 she was awarded the University of Colorado Faculty Book Prize for *Mozart, Westmoreland and Me*. She is a past Director of the Creative Writing Program at University of Colorado, Boulder, and she has served as Artist in Residence at the University of Colorado School of Nursing's Center For Human Caring. She has just completed a novel, *Atomic Open House*.